Fight Fat With Food

Conquer Obesity

With

Smart Diet Choices

Patricia R. McCreary

Table of contents

CHAPTER 10

FIGHTING FAT WITH FOOD: PUTTING IT ALL TOGETHER

Introduction

Melissa had always been an average girl, but her weight had been an issue since she was a child. She was constantly teased and made fun of in school, which only made her feel worse about her weight. She tried to ignore the mocking and bullies, but it was hard to do.

It wasn't until she was in her late teens that she decided to take control of her weight and make a change. She started out by making small changes to her diet and eating habits. She cut out junk food, and sugary snacks, and replaced them with healthier options such as fruit and vegetables. She also began to exercise regularly, going for walks and taking up a sport such as swimming or running.

Melissa was determined to make a difference in her life, and it was paying off. After months of sticking to her new diet and exercise routine, she started to see the results. Her clothes fit better, she had more energy, and she felt better about herself.

But Melissa's journey didn't end there. She knew that the only way to truly conquer her weight issue was to make more permanent lifestyle changes.

She started to focus on portion control, eating smaller meals more often and making sure to get enough sleep each night. She also educated herself on nutrition, learning about the importance of vitamins and minerals in her diet.

By the time Melissa was in her twenties, she had made a complete transformation. She had conquered obesity through smart diet choices and was now living a healthy lifestyle. She was no longer the butt of jokes, but instead a role model for others.

Melissa's story shows that with enough determination and dedication, anything is possible. She proves that it is never too late to make a change and be healthier for yourself.

This is a resource to help you better understand how to use food to improve your health and fight fat. Here, you'll find information on how to make healthy eating a part of your lifestyle, as well as tips and tricks to help you stick to your goals. We'll explore how to create balanced meals, the importance of portion control, and how to make the most out of your grocery shopping trips.

This is the place to come if you're looking to make positive changes to your diet and boost your health. Eating the right foods can help you lose weight, reduce your risk of chronic diseases, and improve your overall well-being.

You don't have to make drastic changes to your diet to see results. Even small tweaks in the way you eat can have a huge impact on your health. With Fight Fat with Food, you'll have the tools and knowledge you need to make those changes and start living a healthier life.

Let's get started on your journey to a healthier you!

Chapter 1

Introduction To Healthy Eating:

Understanding The Basics

Healthy eating is one of the most fundamental components of a healthy lifestyle. Not only does it provide the energy and nutrients we need to survive, but it can also lower our risk of developing chronic diseases, such as obesity, type 2 diabetes, heart disease, and some cancers.

Making healthy food choices is not always easy, especially with the abundance of unhealthy processed and fast foods that are readily available. It is important to understand the basics of healthy eating and how to incorporate it into your daily diet.

To begin, it is important to recognize that there is no one-size-fits-all approach to healthy eating. Everyone's nutritional needs are unique and depend on factors such as age, gender, lifestyle, and activity level. Therefore, it is crucial to consult with a healthcare professional to determine your individual needs and create an eating plan that works for you.

In general, a healthy eating plan should focus on eating a variety of nutrient-dense foods, such as lean proteins, fruits and vegetables, whole grains, and healthy fats. It is also important to limit the consumption of processed and fast foods, as well as foods that are high in saturated fat, salt, and sugar.

A balanced diet does not have to be challenging to consume. Start by selecting a variety of whole foods that you enjoy, and make sure to include foods from each of involving the five dietary groups fruits, vegetables, grains, proteins, and dairy. Try to limit the number of processed foods you eat, and make sure to read nutrition labels to be aware of the ingredients and nutritional content of the foods you choose.

In addition to eating a balanced diet, it is important to establish a regular meal and snack schedule. Eating regularly helps to maintain your energy levels and prevents overeating. It is also important to practice mindful eating, which means being aware of your hunger and fullness cues and paying attention to the flavors and textures of the food you eat.

Finally, it is necessary to be aware of portion sizes. Eating the right amount of food can help you feel satisfied without over-eating.

A good rule of thumb is to fill half of your plate with fruits and vegetables, one-quarter with lean proteins, and one quarter with whole grains.

A healthy lifestyle must include a healthy diet. By understanding the basics of healthy eating and making mindful choices, you can ensure that you are getting all the nutrients you need to stay energized and healthy.

Chapter 2

Understanding Macronutrients: Proteins, Carbohydrates, and Fats

The body's primary energy sources are macronutrients. They include proteins, carbohydrates, and fats. Each macronutrient has a unique role in the body and understanding them is essential for good health.

Proteins are the building blocks of the body. They are made up of amino acids and are responsible for many processes in the body, such as repairing and building tissue, producing hormones, and helping to regulate the immune system. Protein can be found in animal sources such as meat, fish, eggs, and dairy products, as well as in plant sources such as legumes, nuts, and oats.

The body's primary source of energy is carbohydrates. They can be found in foods like grains, fruits, vegetables, dairy products, and legumes. Complex carbohydrates, such as whole grains and legumes, are broken down slowly, providing energy over a longer period of time. Simple carbohydrates, such as sugar and honey, are broken down quickly and provide a rapid source of energy.

Fats are essential for the body, providing energy and helping to absorb vitamins and minerals. Fats can be found in animal sources such as meat, fish, eggs, and dairy products, as well as in plant sources such as nuts, seeds, and avocados. Unsaturated and saturated fats are the two different forms of fats.

Unsaturated fats can be found in foods such as fish and nuts and are considered healthier than saturated fats, which are found in foods such as butter and red meat.

All three macronutrients are necessary for good health. A varied intake of proteins, carbs, and lipids is necessary for a balanced diet. Eating a variety of foods from each food group will help ensure that the body is getting enough of each nutrient. Eating in moderation and exercising regularly will also help to maintain a healthy lifestyle.

Chapter 3

Eating for Weight Loss: Tips and Tricks for a Healthy Diet

Eating for weight loss is an important consideration for people who are looking to make changes to their diet in order to achieve their desired weight loss goals. Eating a healthy diet is essential for weight loss, and there are a few key tips and tricks to help you make the most of your diet.

First and foremost, emphasis should be placed on consuming a balanced diet. Each of the major food groups should be represented by a range of foods in a balanced diet. This includes fruits and vegetables, whole grains, low-fat dairy products, lean proteins, and healthy fats. Eating a variety of foods will help to ensure that you get the vitamins, minerals, and other nutrients that your body needs to function properly.

The second crucial factor is to make sure you are eating enough. Many people who are trying to lose weight can become so focused on cutting calories that they forget to eat enough food. It is important to remember that eating too little can actually have the opposite effect and cause weight gain.

Eating enough food will keep your energy levels up and help to keep your metabolism running smoothly.

Third, it is important to choose nutrient-dense foods. Foods that are packed with nutrients are more filling than those that are low in nutrients. Fruits and vegetables, whole grains, lean meats, and healthy fats are examples of foods that are nutrient-dense. These foods provide your body with the vitamins, minerals, and other nutrients it needs to function properly.

Fourth, Water consumption is crucial. Your body's hydration is crucial for weight loss, and water can help with that.

 Drinking enough water will also help to fill you up and keep your energy levels up.

Finally, it is important to get enough exercise. Exercise helps to burn calories, which can help you lose weight. Set a daily workout goal of at least 30 minutes.

Eating for weight loss is an important part of any diet plan. Following these tips and tricks can help you make the most of your diet, while still getting the nutrients your body needs. Remember, it is important to stay focused on your goals and to be consistent with your diet and exercise plan. With patience and dedication, you can achieve your desired weight loss goals.

Chapter 4

Eating for Energy: How to Balance Your Diet for Optimal Performance

Eating for energy is an important part of maintaining a healthy lifestyle. Our bodies need the right combination of macronutrients, vitamins, and minerals to function at their best and provide us with the energy we need to power through our day. We all know that eating a balanced diet is essential for good health, but how do we ensure that our diet is providing us with the energy we need to stay active and productive?

The key to eating for energy is striking the right balance between macronutrients, vitamins, minerals, and other nutrients. Macronutrients, which include carbohydrates, proteins, and fats, provide our bodies with the energy needed to fuel activities such as physical exercise and cognitive tasks. Carbohydrates are the main source of energy and should make up the majority of our caloric intake.

Proteins, on the other hand, provide our bodies with essential amino acids, which are needed for muscle repair and growth. Fats contain essential fatty acids and are important for hormone production and energy storage.

The right balance of vitamins and minerals is also essential for energy production. Vitamins are essential for many metabolic processes, and the lack of certain vitamins can lead to fatigue and lethargy. The most important vitamins for energy include vitamin B12, which helps convert carbohydrates into energy, and vitamin C, which helps the body absorb iron. Minerals such as iron, zinc, and magnesium are also important for energy production and should be included in a balanced diet.

In addition to macronutrients, vitamins, and minerals, it is also important to include other nutrients in our diets that provide us with energy. These include dietary fiber, which helps regulate the absorption of carbohydrates and keeps us feeling full; antioxidants, which can help protect our cells from damage; and phytonutrients, which provide essential vitamins and minerals.

Finally, when it comes to eating for energy, it is important to practice mindful eating. This means paying attention to how your body feels when you eat and being aware of how different foods affect your energy levels. It also means eating balanced meals that provide your body with the right combination of macronutrients, vitamins, and minerals. Eating regular meals throughout the day is also important, as this will help you to maintain consistent energy levels throughout the day.

In summary, eating for energy is an important part of maintaining a healthy lifestyle. A balanced diet that includes the right combination of macronutrients, vitamins, minerals, and other nutrients is essential for energy production and optimal performance. Eating regular meals and practicing mindful eating can also help you to maintain consistent energy levels throughout the day.

Chapter 5

Eating for Health: Exploring Nutrient-Rich Foods

Eating for health is an important part of overall well-being. Eating a balanced diet that includes nutrient-rich foods helps to nourish your body and provide it with the vitamins and minerals it needs to function properly. Nutrient-rich foods are those that are high in vitamins, minerals, and other essential nutrients while also being low in calories and saturated fats.

Fruits and vegetables are the most nutrient-dense foods available, providing your body with a variety of essential vitamins and minerals. They also include a lot of fiber, which aids in controlling digestion. Examples of nutrient-rich fruits and vegetables include apples, oranges, spinach, sweet potatoes, carrots, and broccoli. Fruits and vegetables are also naturally low in calories, so they can help you maintain a healthy weight.

Whole grains are another important source of nutrients. Whole grains are packed with B vitamins, fiber, and other essential minerals.

Examples of whole-grain foods include oats, brown rice, quinoa, and barley. Eating whole-grain foods can help reduce the risk of heart disease, stroke, and type 2 diabetes.

In addition to fruits and vegetables, seafood is also an excellent source of nutrients. Lean fish such as salmon, tuna, and mackerel are packed with protein and healthy fats. These fish are also high in omega-3 fatty acids, which can help reduce inflammation and improve heart health. Eating fish two to three times per week is recommended for good health.

Dairy products, such as milk and yogurt, are also nutrient-rich foods. Calcium is a key component of dairy products and is necessary for healthy bones and teeth. Dairy products also contain protein, which helps build and maintain muscle, and Vitamin A, which helps promote healthy skin and vision.

Eating a variety of nutrient-rich foods can help ensure that you are receiving the essential vitamins and minerals your body needs. While it is important to eat a balanced diet, it is also important to remember that it is possible to get too much of certain nutrients, such as sodium and saturated fat. Eating too much of these can lead to health problems, such as high blood pressure and heart disease. For this reason, it is important to read nutrition labels and avoid foods that are high in sodium or saturated fat.

By eating a variety of nutrient-rich foods, you can provide your body with the essential vitamins and minerals it needs to stay healthy and strong. Eating nutritious foods can also help you maintain a healthy weight and reduce the risk of certain diseases. So make sure to include a variety of nutrient-rich foods in your diet to get the most nutritional benefit.

CHAPTER 6

Mindful Eating: How to Listen to Your Body's Signals

Mindful eating is a mindful practice that allows us to be aware of our physical and emotional sensations related to food. It is a way of being present and aware of the experience of eating, rather than being distracted or absent. This practice can help us to become more aware of our body's signals, recognize when we are truly hungry, and to choose foods that are best for our physical and mental well-being.

The goal of mindful eating is to become more in tune with our body's signals, to recognize when we are truly hungry, and to choose foods that are best for our physical and mental well-being. Mindful eating is not a diet; it is an approach to eating that can help us to be more conscious and aware of our choices and to create a healthier relationship with food.

One way to begin is to practice mindful eating before, during, and after meals.

Before a meal, take a few moments to check in with your body and assess your hunger level. Are you truly hungry, or are you eating out of habit or in response to emotions? During a meal, take time to savor each bite. Notice the taste, texture, and smell of your food. Chew slowly to allow your digestive system to signal your brain that you are full. After a meal, check in with yourself and assess if you are satisfied or if you need more.

Mindful eating also involves paying attention to what is going on around you. Are you eating in a hurry or a relaxed environment? Are you surrounded by distractions like the television or your phone? Taking the time to be mindful of your environment can help to create a more mindful eating experience.

Finally, mindful eating involves being aware of the emotional and physical sensations that come with food. Some foods can give us an emotional boost, while others can make us feel sluggish. Paying attention to these sensations can help us to make better food choices.

Mindful eating is a practice that can help us to become more aware of our body's signals and to create a healthier relationship with food. Taking the time to practice mindful eating before, during, and after meals and to be aware of our environment and our emotions can help us to make better food choices and to become more in tune with our body's needs.

Chapter 7

Eating for Longevity: How to Make Nutrition Choices for Long-Term Health

When it comes to longevity and health, nutrition plays an integral role. Eating for longevity is about making smart nutritional choices that will benefit your body both now and in the long run. Eating for longevity is about choosing health-promoting foods that will provide your body with the essential nutrients it needs to stay healthy and strong.

Let's start by discussing some of the key components of eating for longevity. The first step is to eat a balanced diet that includes a variety of nutrient-dense foods. Fruits and vegetables are excellent sources of vitamins, minerals, fiber, and other essential nutrients. Whole grains, legumes, lean proteins, and healthy fats are also important components of a healthy diet. Eating a variety of these foods will help ensure that you get a broad range of essential nutrients to support your body's needs.

The second step is to limit or avoid processed and refined foods. Processed and refined foods are typically high in calories, fat, and sugar, and low in essential nutrients. These foods can contribute to weight gain, chronic diseases, and other health problems. Instead, focus on eating whole, unprocessed foods like fruits, vegetables, nuts, seeds, and whole grains.

The next phase entails being mindful of portion sizes. Eating too much of any food can lead to weight gain and an increased risk of chronic diseases. Approximately half of your meal should consist of fruits and vegetables, with the other half being made up of lean proteins and healthy fats. Stick to smaller portions of higher-calorie and higher-fat foods.

The fourth step is to be mindful of your eating habits. Mindful eating is about being aware of your body's hunger and fullness cues and making intentional choices about what and how much you eat. Eating slowly and taking time to enjoy your food can help you to be more mindful of your eating habits.

Finally, make sure you stay hydrated. Drinking enough water is essential for good health. Try to drink 8 to 10 glasses of water each day. Water can help to keep your body hydrated, fill you up, and prevent overeating.

Eating for longevity is about making smart nutrition choices that will benefit your body both now and in the long run. Choosing nutrient-dense whole foods, limiting or avoiding processed and refined foods, paying attention to portion sizes, being mindful of your eating habits, and drinking plenty of water can help you to make healthy nutrition choices that will promote long-term health.

Chapter 8

The Role of Exercise in Weight Loss and Health

When it comes to weight loss and health, exercise plays a major role. Exercise can not only help you lose weight, but also improve your overall health, mental well-being, and quality of life.

Exercise helps you lose weight by burning calories. When you exercise, your body needs to use energy to move, and that energy comes from the food you eat, which is typically stored as fat. When the energy you use is greater than the energy you consume, your body will break down fat to use as energy, resulting in weight loss.

Exercise also helps you maintain a healthy weight. Regular physical activity helps your body to use energy more efficiently. This means that you will burn more calories even when you're not exercising, resulting in an overall reduction in body fat.

In addition to helping you lose weight and maintain a healthy weight, exercise also offers numerous health benefits.

Regular physical activity can help reduce your risk of many chronic diseases, such as heart disease, stroke, and diabetes. It can also help reduce stress and anxiety, improve your mood, and even help you sleep better.

Finally, exercise can improve your quality of life. Regular physical activity can help you feel more energetic and improve your self-esteem. It can also help you stay connected to friends and family since physical activity is often a great way to socialize.

Many different types of exercise can help you lose weight and improve your health. Finding a hobby or something you enjoy and can do frequently is the key. Some popular options include walking, running, biking, swimming, weight training, and yoga.

The amount of exercise you need to lose weight and improve your health varies from person to person. Generally, the American College of Sports Medicine recommends at least 150 minutes of moderate-intensity physical activity each week. This can be divided into five, thirty-minute sessions each day. However, if you're just starting, you may want to start slowly and gradually work up to more intense activities.

Regardless of the workout you select, it's critical to maintain motivation.

Set realistic goals, track your progress, and reward yourself when

you reach those goals. Exercise can be hard work, but it's worth it

in the end!

Chapter 9

Building Healthy Habits: Learning to Love Healthy Living

Building healthy habits is essential to living a long and healthy life. We all know that eating right and exercising regularly is important, but there are many other habits that are equally important. Learning to love healthy living is a process, but with a little guidance and commitment, you can develop healthy habits that will help you stay healthy for years to come.

The first step in building healthy habits is to create an environment that encourages healthy behaviors. This means removing unhealthy snacks from your kitchen, signing up for a gym membership, or simply scheduling regular walks with a friend. Having a plan in place and setting realistic goals will help you stay focused on your health goals.

The next step is to create a routine that includes these healthy activities. Make sure to schedule your workouts, healthy meals, and relaxation activities into your daily routine. This will help you make healthy habits a part of your everyday lifestyle.

Additionally, it's critical to spice up your routine. This could include trying different types of exercise, exploring new recipes, or even taking up a new hobby. Variety helps keep you motivated and excited about healthy living.

In addition to developing healthy habits, it is also important to build positive relationships with others. Having a strong support system of family and friends who understand and encourage your healthy lifestyle can help you stay on track. It is also important to find an accountability partner who can help you stay motivated and stick to your goals.

Finally, it is important to remember that building healthy habits takes time. It is a procedure that calls for persistence and dedication. If you are feeling overwhelmed, start small and focus on one healthy habit at a time. Start by including more fruits and vegetables in your diet, for instance. Once that becomes a habit, you can add other healthy habits such as regular exercise or replace unhealthy snacks with healthier options.

Learning to love healthy living can be a challenge, but it is worth the effort. With commitment and dedication, you can build healthy habits that will last a lifetime.

Chapter 10

Fighting Fat with Food: Putting It All Together

Fighting fat with food is a great way to improve your overall health and well-being, as well as lose weight. The key is to eat the right types of food and ensure you get enough of the essential nutrients your body needs. Planning ahead and making smart food choices can help you stay on track.

First, consider the types of food you should eat. Eating a balanced diet is important, and that means including a variety of food groups in your meals. Focus on lean proteins such as fish and poultry, whole grains, fruits and vegetables, low-fat dairy products, and healthy fats like olive oil, avocado, and nuts.

Second, make sure you're getting enough of the essential nutrients your body needs. Vitamins, minerals, and essential fatty acids are essential for your body to function properly.

Some of the most important nutrients include fiber, calcium, iron, vitamin A, and vitamin C. Eating a variety of foods can help ensure you get enough of these important nutrients.

Third, portion control is key when it comes to fighting fat with food. Weight gain can occur even when eating nutritious meals in excess. It's crucial to calculate and adhere to your portion sizes. You can also try to make healthier choices by replacing high-calorie snacks with healthier alternatives, such as nuts, fruits, or vegetables.

Finally, it's important to stay hydrated. Water consumption throughout the day can significantly reduce hunger and cravings. It can also help flush out toxins and keep your body functioning optimally.

In conclusion, fighting fat with food is an important part of achieving a healthy weight and improving your overall health. Eating a variety of healthy foods and making sure you get enough of the essential nutrients your body needs can help you lose weight and maintain your health. Additionally, portion control and drinking plenty of water are important parts of maintaining a healthy weight. By following these tips, you can achieve your weight loss goals and maintain a healthy body.

9 798391 503446